Preface

I do not profess to be the expert in bodyweight exercises. I am just a busy professional, married with three daughters who has been there and done that, learning and achieving respectable results in the process. There is a lot of information on the subject out there. Through this book it is my hope to share my experience and what I have learnt in the process as concisely and easy to follow as possible.

Contents

The Why?

Matt is a busy professional. When he was younger, he enjoyed being active in sports. During weekends he would frequent the gym, play table-tennis at a local club, swim and sprint. However after graduating from university and now married with three lovely daughters, priorities had changed. At a height of 5 feet 6 inches and weight of 80 kilogrammes, Matt was not the fittest. His cholesterol and blood pressure levels became borderline high. Energy was low. Occasional neck and backaches made things worse.

Something had to change. Apart from career goals, Matt now wanted to stay healthy for his family. He got to know about calisthenics or body-weight exercise from the internet a year and a half ago. After plenty of research, he finally embarked on his journey. Fast forward to today, he is now down to 68 kilogrammes with 15 percent body fat. Cholesterol and blood pressure levels are now in check. No more neck or backaches. He can now keep up with his three children. In fact, work efficiency has improved as he can concentrate and focus better.

Regardless of what exercise 'vehicle' it may be, the most important driver is the 'why' and not the 'how'. It is hardest in the beginning as there will be a new routine. The 'why' will motivate you to keep things going. Once the initial phase has been overcome and a new habit has been instilled, exercise becomes fun rather than a chore. This usually takes about a month. 'Happy' hormones are secreted by the body into the blood circulation during exercise. Additionally, the production of 'repair' and 'healing' hormones is vamped up after a consistent 2-3 months of exercise. This is when changes in strength and body physique become obvious. Exercise then turns addictive.

Matt chose calisthenics as it is very flexible and is not equipment intensive. Calisthenics can be done practically anywhere. You just need your bodyweight. The rest is all imagination and creativity. You do not need to subscribe to expensive gym memberships. Don't get me wrong. Going to the gym to workout is beneficial and wonderful. However Matt did not want to dress up, travel down, do his workout and then come home. He even sometimes does his workouts in his pyjamas. Sometimes even the thought of making an effort to travel puts one off. Calisthenics can be done in the comfort of your own home or your neighbourhood park if you want to.

In fact, one can easily tailor the programmes to fit ones needs and schedule. No peak periods or taking turns to use the bench press. However Matt did have to learn a few basic principles. Of course there were techniques he had to fine tune and correct along the way. And he is still learning and improving. The learning never stops!

Some basic principles

For all forms of weight-training there are a few basic principles which apply.

1) **In general, the number of repetitions to failure (when you are unable to complete a full repetition) concentrates more on a particular goal.**

Strength: 2-4 repetitions

Mass: 6-12 repetitions

Tone and endurance: 20 or more repetitions

For example if one can perform a push-up 7 times till failure this would encourage more muscle growth. Of course there will be some element of strength and endurance gains but the gains would mainly be that for mass. This also holds true for low repetitions of 2-4 which would focus on building strength and less on mass. High repetitions (20 or more) are good for toning and endurance but less so for strength and building mass. As such adjust your intensity and thence repetitions accordingly to meet your goals. For each exercise perform 3-5 sets with 2 minutes of rest in between.

2) **Ideally each muscle group should be trained twice a week.**

The old adage 'use it or lose it' holds true for weight-training. Two times a week works best to stimulate and maintain muscle growth. The key word here is ideally. If your schedule does not permit that, then once a week is the minimum. The body is a very efficient machine. What the body feels it does not need, it will get rid of. Unutilised muscle fibres will be removed. This allows the body to conserve metabolic requirements and focus on where the demand lies. When stimulated, the muscle growth factors kick into action once again. Increasing the size and density of muscle takes much longer than decreasing them. Therefore it is best to keep to a regular programme for maintenance at least.

3) Varying the type or intensity of exercise confuses the muscles and leads to more gains.

Matt knows that after a while the body accommodates and adapts. After 6 months of exercise Matt faced stagnating gains and plateaus in strength increase. This is fine if the aim is to maintain and keep fit. However, Matt wanted some more gains. Hence he made some minor tweaks to his programme every 6 months and things started rolling again. A change in the intensity and the type of exercise although involving the same group of muscles confuses them; a term called muscle confusion. When muscle is confused, it does only one thing – grow. The good news is, these tweaks do not need to be major. Just a simple change perhaps in speed, rhythm or sets is enough for confusion. You do not necessarily have to overhaul your programme. But you can always do that if you want to – it just takes a little creativity.

4) Proper technique is key.

a) Posture and movement

When first starting out, it is vital to learn the correct posture and movement. This not only optimises the effectiveness of the workout but also prevents injuries. As such begin with a low intensity. In other words if you cannot do more than 12 repetitions for a particular exercise, lower the intensity. Starting off right prevents damage and injuries in the long run. Additionally, you would be able to develop a better mind muscle connection earlier on.

b) Mind muscle connection

This is exactly what it is. It is the conscious activation of the relevant muscle intended and not merely just finishing the repetition. This prevents the occasional 'cheating' where a repetition is performed inadequately or wrongly. Mind muscle connection goes hand in hand with achieving a better posture and movement - ultimately leading to better technique and performance. For instance when working out the chest muscles also known as the pectoralis major let us say during a push-up, one should think about the muscle contracting, then squeezing the muscle at the top of the movement then relaxing and finally feel and concentrate on the stretch. Of course other muscles will be at work for a push-up but you get my point. An appreciation of the mind muscle concentration avoids bouncing and allows a stricter form. In addition, it fatigues and stimulates the muscles more effectively providing for a more fruitful workout.

c) Use the full range of motion

Utilising the entire range of motion for a particular exercise recruits as many muscle fibres as possible. By this I mean going from a full stretch of a muscle through to the full contraction – hence giving a greater workout. Although you might not be able to do this all the time, there are sometimes simple ways around it. For example, a full stretch of the chest muscles is limited by the floor during a push-up. You can overcome this by elevating yourself on furniture say chairs to clear the body from the floor. Matt bought a set of parallettes which are like handle bars placed on the floor to increase the distance of the chest from the floor.

d) **Don't neglect the negatives**

It pays to pay attention to the negatives. The 'negative' is simply the phase of the repetition where there is controlled relaxation. The muscles are still working but lengthening at the same time. This phase causes the most microscopic damage to the muscles and so more growth stimuli. Matt has a simple rule of thumb (1-1-3) – 1 second positive, 1 second squeeze, 3 seconds negative. A good push up would be to push up in 1 second, then contracting the chest muscles at the top for 1 second, then slowly drop the chest to the floor over a controlled 3 seconds.

5) Rest and nutrition are just as important

Muscle gains actually occur during rest and not during exercise. Exercise is specifically to stimulate the muscles, to break them down, to tell them they need to develop. The healing, repair and hypertrophy (increase in size) of the muscle fibre happen while sleeping and relaxing. Not giving the muscle enough time to recover and adapt is counter-intuitive. The actual workout performance deteriorates. Matt found out the hard way. He was not only stagnating but the number of solid repetitions decreased. Now realising that rest is equally important, Matt does not work the same body part earlier than two days. This has translated into better strength and mass gains.

Body tissue requires building blocks. For muscle, its main constituent is amino acids – protein. Matt subscribes to the 1 gram per pound of body-weight per day (1g/lb/day). He tries to keep to lean meat like fish and chicken. But he does pamper himself from time to time. In addition to this, minerals and vitamins are needed to complete the healing and metabolism of tissue. Hence an ideal diet would also consist of plenty of fruit and vegetables. Matt takes his 5 servings per day religiously. He likes green-leafy vegetables and tomatoes. His favourite fruits include papayas, bananas, oranges, kiwis and mangoes. Matt keeps a jar of mixed nuts on his desk at work for snacks.

The benefits of having a little more muscle

Matt's initial intention when starting calisthenics was to lose weight, improve his health and to stay fit for his family. Some of the benefits of gaining muscle include:

1) **Brain power**

Matt found that he now can concentrate and focus more during work. His attention span and memory have also benefitted. This is more of an indirect effect of gaining muscle, through better oxygenation and blood circulation due to the regular exercise.

2) **Bone health**

Although not always the case, but stronger muscles by and large also mean stronger bones. In the midst of weight-training, the human skeleton is loaded. For a normal healthy person Wolff's law applies (bone will adapt to the loads under which it is placed). The bone will remodel or change its architecture over time to be able to resist greater loads. In other words the bone will thicken and become denser. Unfortunately, the converse is true. Stop loading the bone and it will become thinner and weaker. This phenomenon was seen in the very first astronauts on returning from space where they sustained fragility fractures. This was a result of the lack of gravity in space which caused a decrease in bone mass. Hence now astronauts need to regularly use elastic resistance bands for exercise to maintain their bone mass whilst in space.

3) **Cardiovascular health**

Weight-training will raise your heart rate and make it pump harder. Do this regularly and this would be just what the doctor prescribed. The heart will be healthier and pump more efficiently. Blood flow will also be smoother. Furthermore, it will boost your high-density lipoprotein (your "good" cholesterol) and decrease unhealthy low-density lipoprotein levels. This reduces the risk of getting a heart attack or even a stroke.

4) **Coordination**

Calisthenics athletes move their own body in space and time. Constant practise of technique and mind muscle connection develops functional strength as well. This benefit is advantageous and transferable to other fields of sports because the body is the weight being controlled and not an artificial weight. At the same time excellent control and proprioception (position sense) enhances coordination.

5) **Easier fat loss**

Fat is one of the ways the body stores excess energy. This is converted back to carbohydrates or ketones in times of demand leading to 'fat-loss'. Exercise helps burn fat when the demand exceeds supply. Muscle tissue uses up a lot of energy not only to function but to be built and to survive. As such there is greater metabolism and energy demand even at rest. This aids fat loss but only if there is a net negative balance. If intake of calories increases and exceeds the loss, this would only lead to a positive balance and thence fat gain.

6) Energy

With a more efficient heart pump, blood circulation and oxygenation of body tissues, one would feel more energised. As the body gets stronger, work output is greater and less susceptible to fatigue. The mind is also more refreshed and efficient which translates to more restful sleep and focused work done.

7) Less stress

Exercise releases the hormone "endorphin" which not only has a reward effect but also a 'feel good' component. This puts the body and mind into a more relaxed state. In stressful states the body and mind function less optimally for everyday chores or work as the goal is to prepare for 'flight or fight' like when a wild animal approaches. On the contrary a relaxed state allows the body to conserve energy and drive it towards your work, be it writing a speech or preparing a project report. Apart from that stress hormone levels are kept at bay, keeping blood vessels more relaxed and blood pressure in check over the long term.

What Matt does

Matt tries to work each body part twice a week. Of course his work schedule does not always permit that. But that is okay. He will then just pick up where he left off and continue at the first chance he can. This means that if he stops at chest, then he will continue on with legs the next time round. His regular is routine is as such:

Day 1 - Back and biceps

Day 2 – Chest, shoulders, triceps

Day 3 – Legs

Day 4 – Back and biceps

Day 5 – Chest, shoulders, triceps

Day 6 - Legs

Day 7 – Rest

Matt has a confession. He dislikes working on his abdominal muscles. As you can see he does not have an ab day. The good news is that calisthenics exercises utilises compound movements. As such every exercise day is also an ab day. Of course if you have the time and dedication to, please incorporate some abdominal workout into your routines. These include crutches, leg raises, planks, dragonflags and so forth.

Day 1 ('Pull day') – Back and biceps

For this Matt loves the pull-up. This focuses on the back muscles, the latissimus dorsi and the biceps brachii. The trapezius and the posterior deltoids also get a slight workout. Matt adds a slight tweak to this by combining an isometric (contracting the muscle but not changing its length) leg-raise.

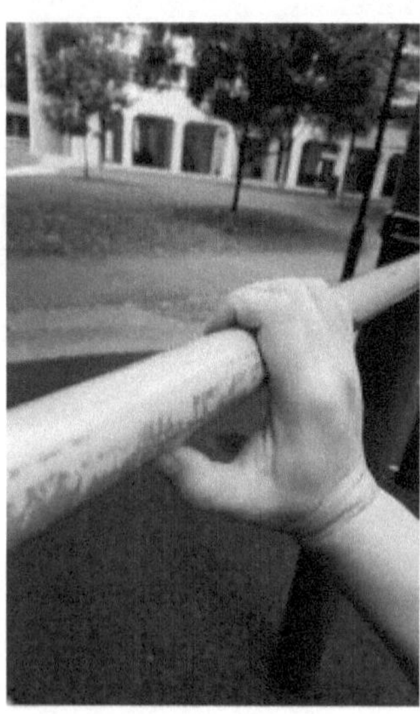
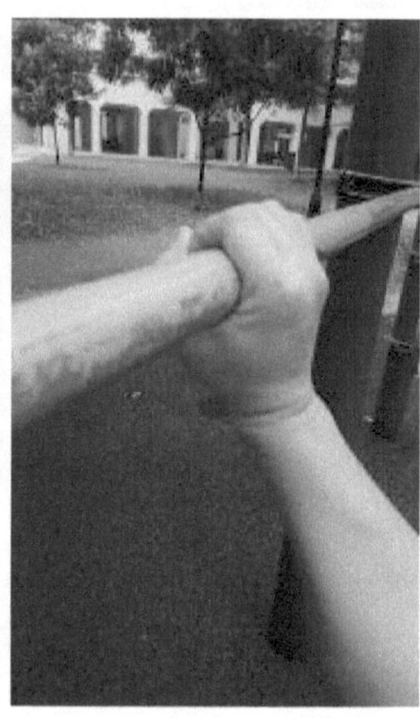

Figure 1a. The grip. Hook the bar with your hands rather than wrap around it. Matt discovered this the hard way. By trying to wrap his palms around the bar, the hands will slide down slightly during the pull up and cause focal pressure areas leading to thick calluses (hard, raised skin). Matt now hooks the bar, find that resting position where the palm does not roll downwards then complete his full grip. Of course he still has calluses but these are small and not super thick and peeling.

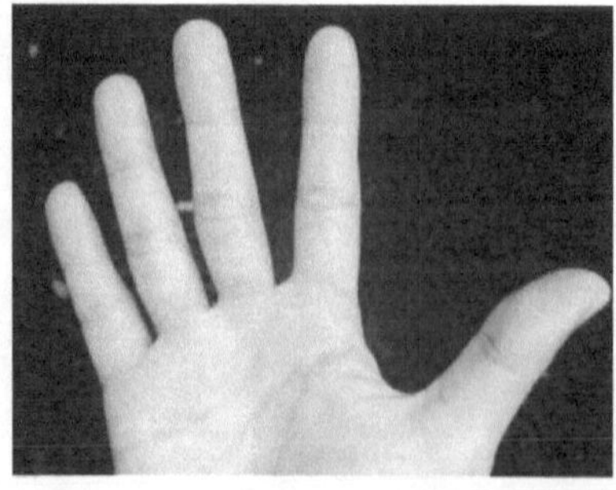

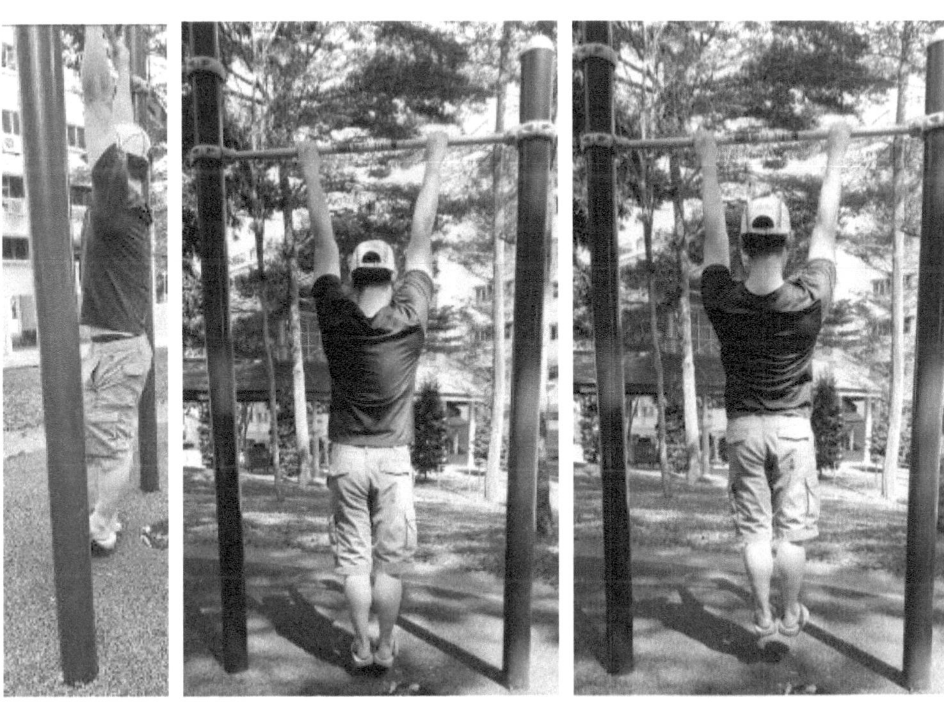

Figure 1b. Scapula (shoulder blade) depresses. Now Matt uses this first set as a warm up to brace his shoulder joints. Instead of the full pull-up he lets his body hang then depresses his shoulder blades. Hands slightly more than shoulder width apart. Palms facing forward. Squeeze the buttocks to keep the legs stiff and contract the abdominal muscles. The entire core is now recruited and the body rigid to prevent swinging during the pull-up which gives a bad form and reduces the effectiveness of the workout. Matt also gets a good core exercise with this! 12 repetitions are sufficient.

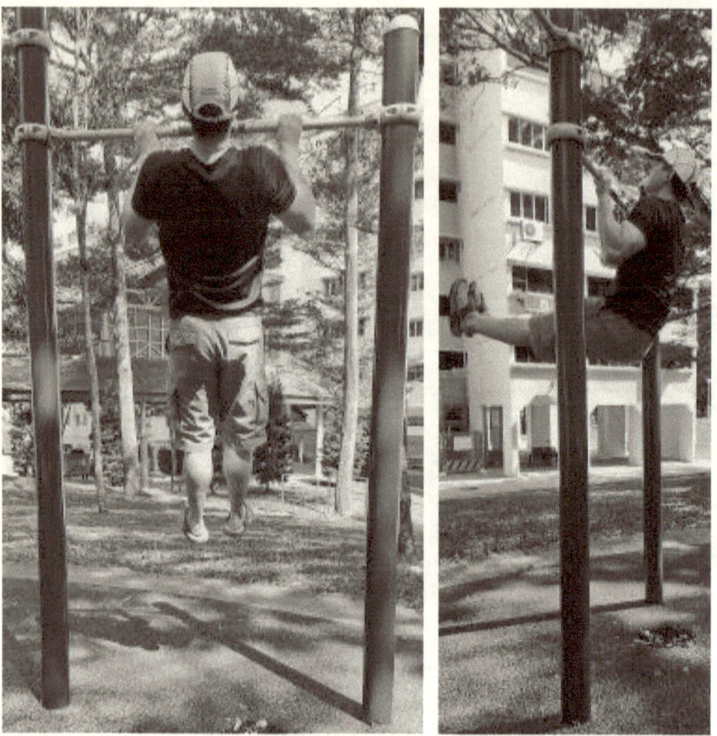

Figure 1c. Now for the second set. Pull-up till the chin is above the bar. However instead on concentrating on getting the chin above the bar, Matt finds that concentrating on pulling his chest to the bar gives a better contraction of his back muscles. In addition before starting the pull-up, Matt elevates his legs in full extension so that they are parallel to the ground and keeps them in this position throughout the set. This gives the abdominal muscles a workout at the same time.

At the top, Matt tries to squeeze his elbows together like clasping his chest wall with his elbows. He then holds it for a second then slowly goes down to the bottom over 3 seconds. After one and a half years of training Matt can do 14 pull ups with correct form. But he does not stop there, he will still try to continue with more repetitions although with incomplete range, till he is unable to bear with the muscle burn then stop.

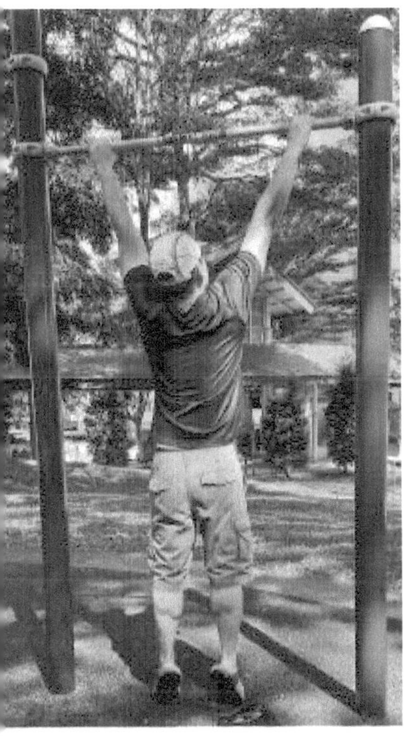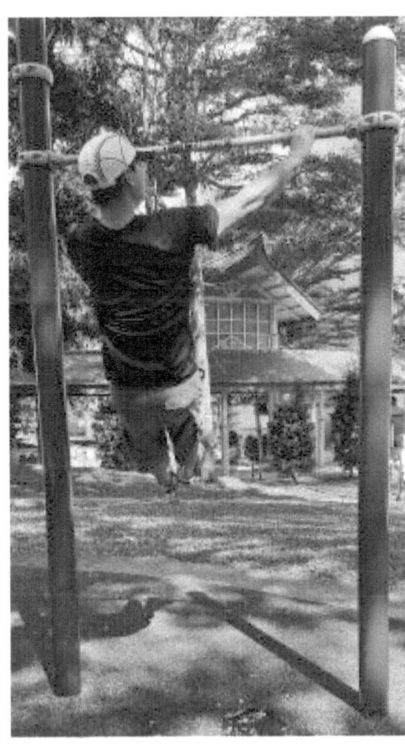

Figure 1d. For the third set, Matt does the 'Archer' pull-up. For this, he pulls with only one arm while the other arm is kept straight but with the grip still on the bar. He is only able to do 3-4 on each side. Then quickly continues with the pull-up till failure. This routine of dropping the intensity without the regular rest interval is called a 'drop-set'.

For the fourth set, Matt does the chin-up. Instead of palms facing forwards, they now face backwards and are directly in front of the shoulders respectively. Although all these exercise use more or less the same muscle groups, the pull-up uses more latissimus dorsi power while the chin-up, more biceps brachii power. The wide grip pull-up further uses more latissimus dorsi power and less that of the biceps.

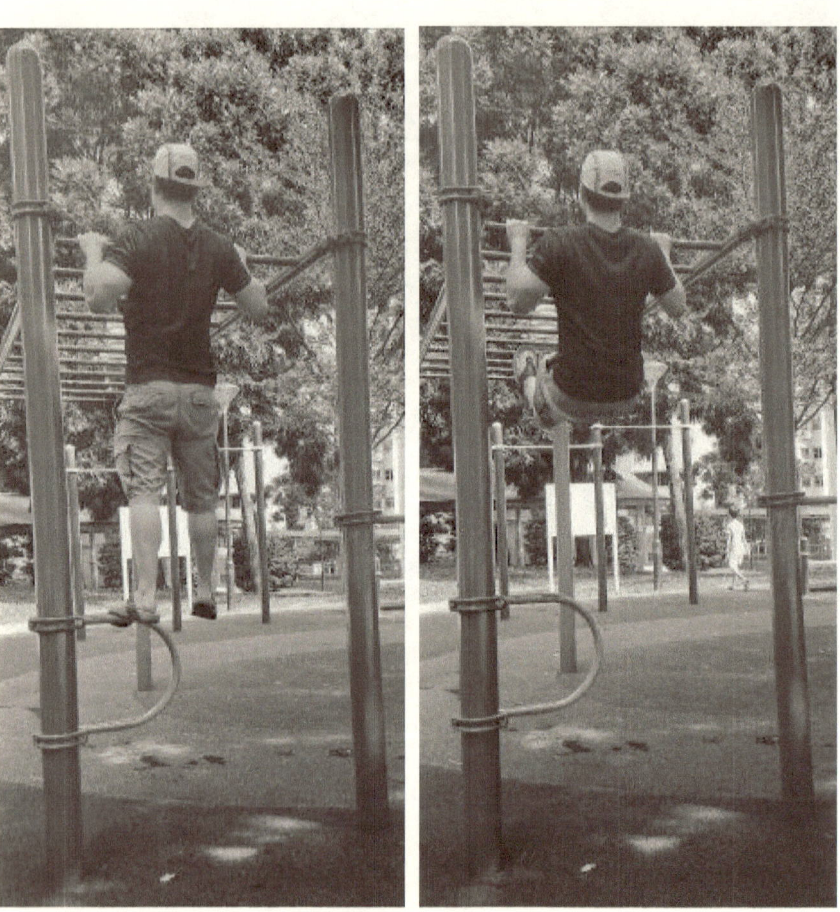

Figure 1e. Matt initially started doing negatives and 'Australian' pull-ups as he could not do a single pull-up repetition. Matt would still warm-up with the scapula depresses. But then start his repetition at the top and slowly lower himself in a controlled manner over 3 seconds. Do not look down on the negatives as they are equally important for muscle and strength development.

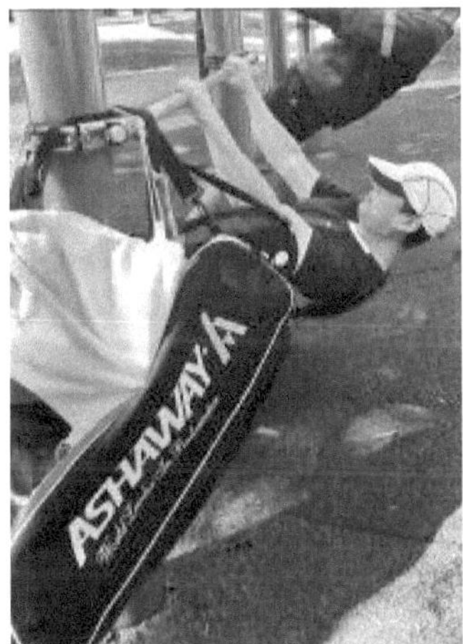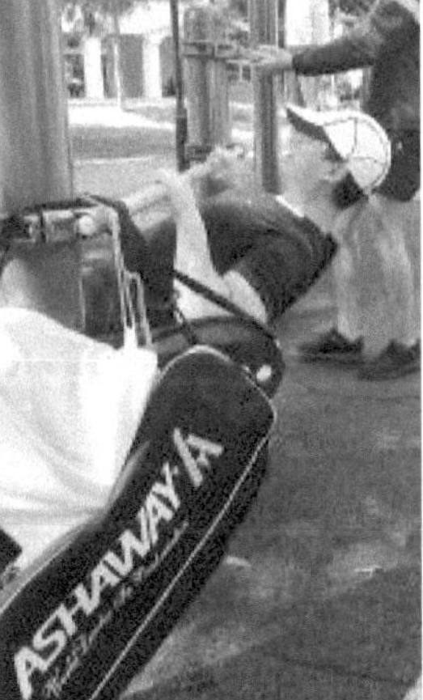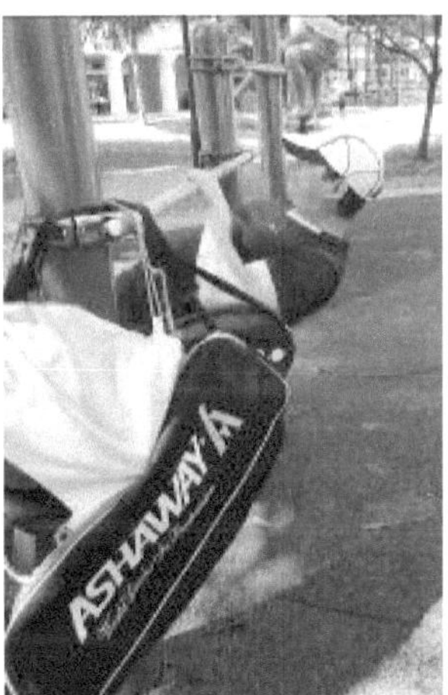

Figure 1f. This pull up variation was given the name 'Australian' pull-up as you start 'down under' the bar in a more horizontal position. This variation is easier as the weight of the body is partially supported by the ground. Again, make sure your buttocks and abdominal muscles are squeezed tight. Adjust so that with a complete pull the bar is just at the nipple line. You can later progress this to the one-arm 'Australian' pull-up.

In summary

)   Correct grip, hand slightly more than shoulder width apart, rigid body

i)   1st set scapula (shoulder blade) depresses: 12 reps

ii)   2nd set pull-ups: Till failure

v)   3rd set archer pull-ups: Till failure then drop-set pull-ups to failure

)   4th set chin-ups: Till failure

         (if unable to perform at least 6 proper repetitions of the pull-up, start with the

         negatives and the 'Australian' pull-up to build up strength)

Day 2 ("Push day") – Chest, shoulders, triceps

The push-up is Matt's favourite for working these muscles. The muscles involved include the pectoralis muscles, deltoids and triceps brachii.

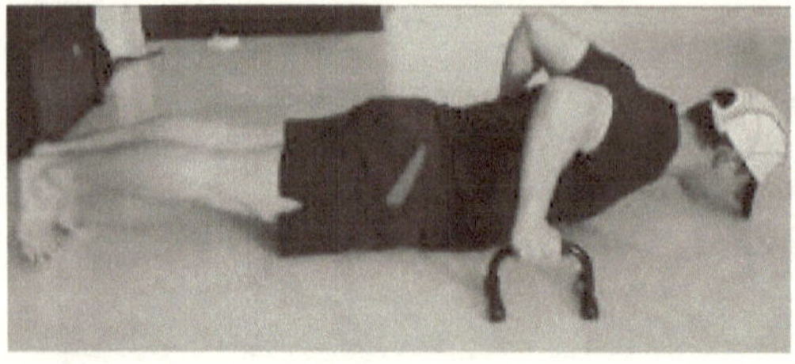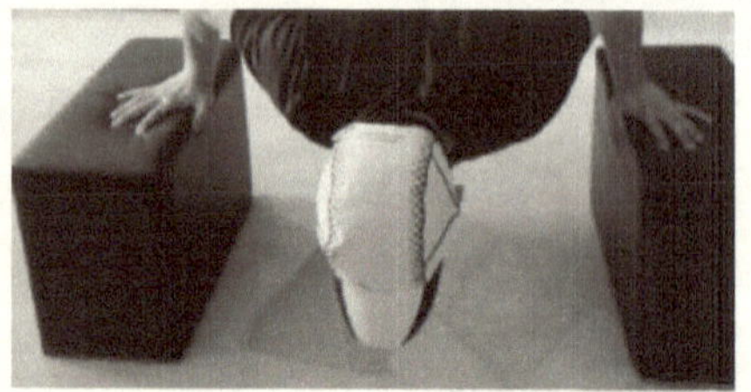

Figure 2a. You start by lying chest down on the floor with palms at shoulder width apart and thumbs at nipple height. Again you want your body to be rigid – squeeze your buttocks and tighten your abdominal muscles.

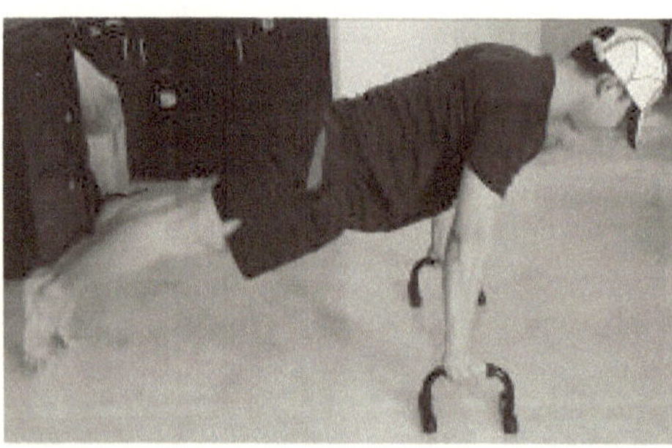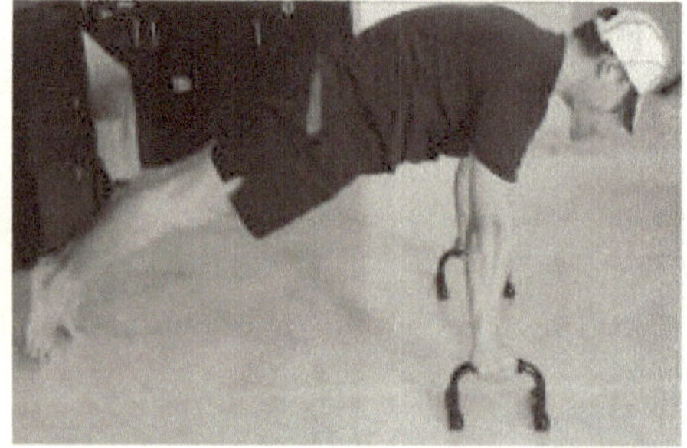

Figure 2b. Push your body to the top. But don't stop there. Push the shoulder blades forward (scapula protraction) and squeeze the chest muscles together. The scapula protraction concentrates on the serratus anterior – the strip like muscle at the sides of the abdominal muscle just below the chest muscles.

Matt realized that he is unable to achieve a full stretch of the chest muscles on descending. Although not compulsory, Matt prefers to use parallettes (small low handle bars) which he bought off the internet (previously Matt used his coffee-table stools for this). In this way the floor no longer limits his descend before reaching a full stretch of the chest muscles, hence allowing him to use the full range of the muscle and perform a more effective workout.

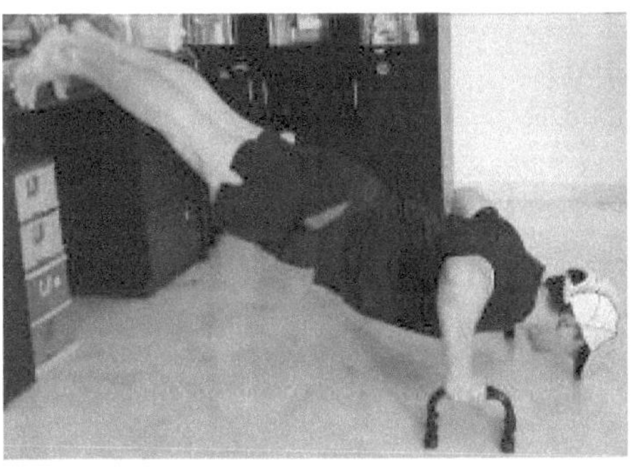 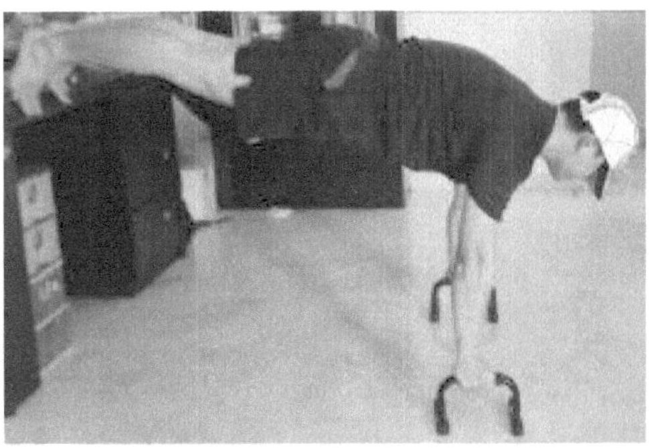

Figure 2c. Decline push-up. After doing about 30 repetitions as a warm-up, Matt elevates his feet on his study desk while his hands kept on the parallettes on the floor (decline push-ups). This increases the effective weight. However because of the new angle it does work more of the upper chest and shoulder. Matt is able to do 20 repetitions then quickly drops down to do regular push-ups till failure then push-up on his knees instead of on the feet till failure. This is his second set.

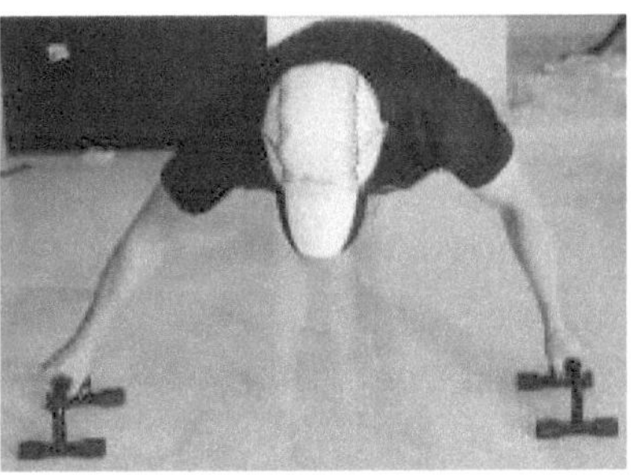 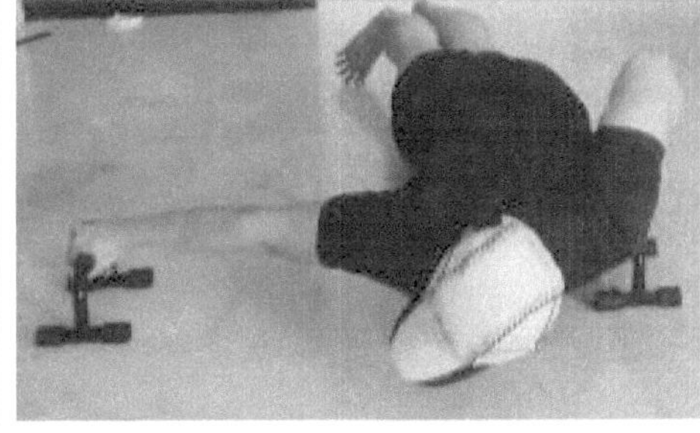

Figure 2d. Decline 'Archer' push-ups. For this Matt keeps his feet elevated on the study table, hands on the parallettes. The hands are now no longer at shoulders' width apart but about an additional hand's breadth wider from the shoulders. Matt now shifts the body so that the same side chest is just above the hand while the other arm is kept straight. For example, left chest over left hand with the right arm kept straight (adjust the width of the hands apart to accommodate for this). Push-up with the single left arm, then shift to the right side and repeat. Matt is able to perform 6 repetitions on each side. Again once done to failure, Matt quickly drops

his legs down to the floor and performs the standard push-up on parallettes followed by push-ups on the knees till failure.

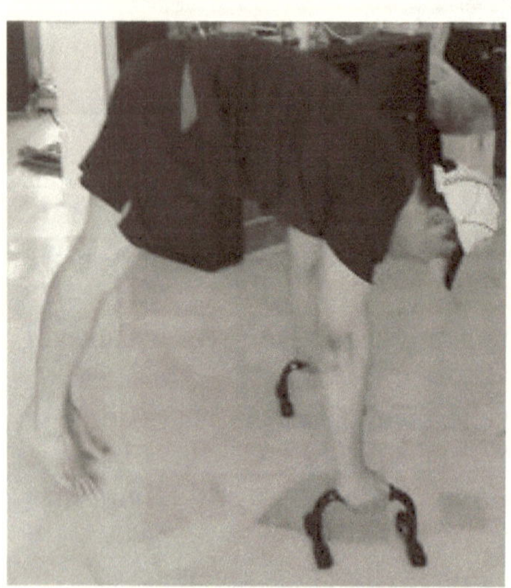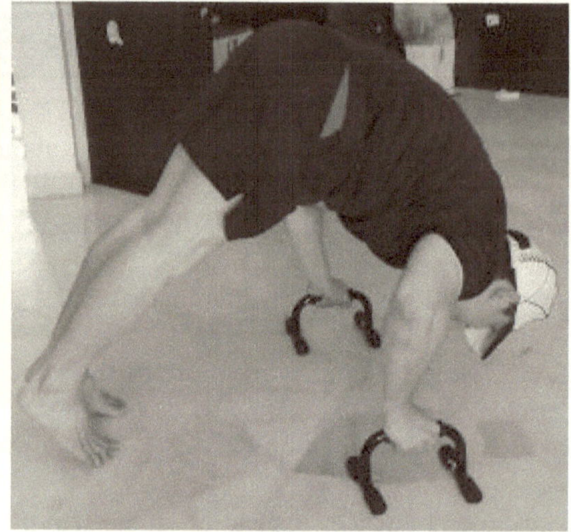

Figure 2e. The 'Pike' push-up. This exercise concentrates more on the shoulders. Matt uses the parallettes for this exercise as well to take advantage of the full stretch and range of motion. The hands are placed slightly more than shoulder width apart. Now bend down towards the floor flexing at the hips. The body will now be in an inverted jack-knife position like an upside down letter 'V'. How close should the feet be to the hands? Matt will be on tip-toes and lean over so that he can feel the weight of the body entirely over his palms and almost going to tip over. He slowly lowers his head as much as he can over 3 seconds and even extends his head backwards to give extra space to clear the floor. Then pushes up over a second and squeezes his shoulder muscles for one second before going on to the next repetition. Matt does about 12 repetitions.

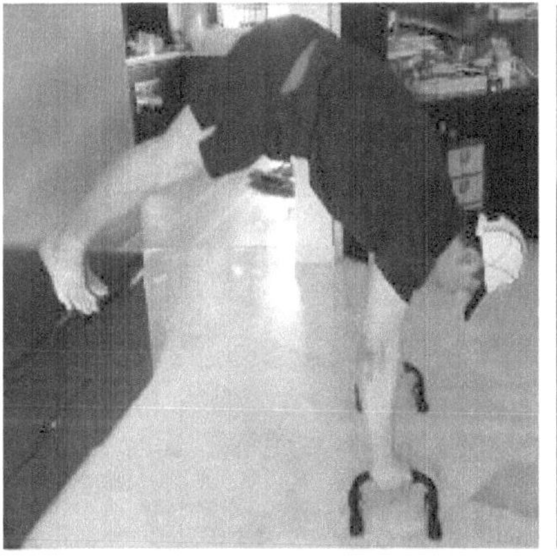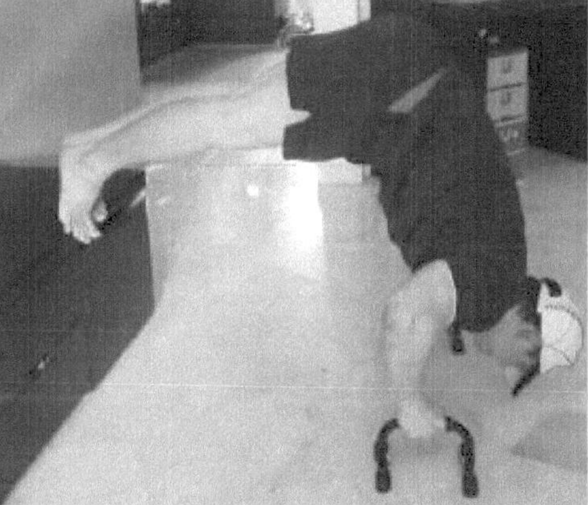

Figure 2f. The 'Pike' push-up with feet elevated. Matt places his feet on his coffee-table for this. However do note that there is a risk of tipping over as you descend. So adjust the distance of your hands from your feet accordingly. Do 12 repetitions. Matt has been trying to practise the hand-stands but it still unable to achieve balance. He previously did handstands against the wall but prefers to do the 'Pike' push-ups instead. Matt then finishes off with another regular 'Pike' push-up till failure and then quickly drops set to the regular push-up till failure.

In summary

.)   Hands shoulder width apart, body rigid

i)   1st set: push-up on parallettes till failure

ii)   2nd set: decline push-up on paralletes till failure then drop-set to regular push-ups then push-up on knees till failure

v)   3rd set: decline 'Archer' push-up on parallettes till failure then regular push-ups then push-up on knees till failure

v)   4th set: 'Pike' push-ups till failure

vi)   5th set: Elevated 'Pike' push-ups till failure

vii)   6th set: 'Pike' push-ups till failure then drop-set to push-ups till failure

Day 3 (Leg-day): Gluteus muscles, Quadriceps, Hamstrings, Calf

Do not neglect your lower limb exercises. The legs are just as important especially for functional strength or sports as they propel the body in space and support the entire body when lifting or pushing a heavy object. Just like the core muscles, you will feel the legs getting a mild workout during the Day 1 and Day 2 exercises. This is because of the fact that calisthenics is a very functional form of workout and still recruits and engages these other muscles during the exercise routines in order to stabilise the body.

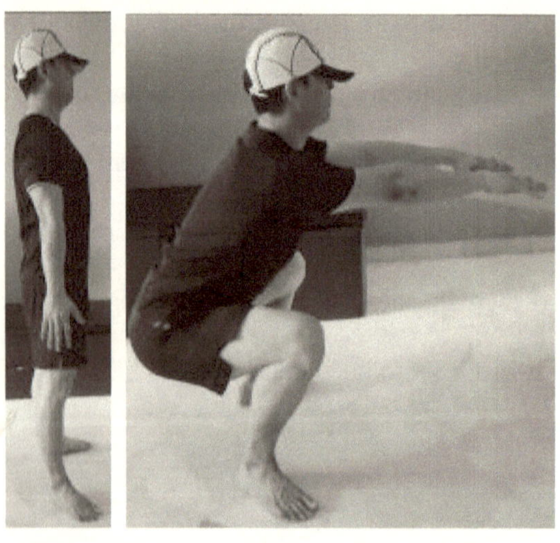

Figure 3a. Squats. This works more of the quadriceps and gluteus muscles. Matt uses this as his warm-up set. Stand straight with feet shoulder width apart. Tighten your core. Matt faces his study desk clock to time himself. Get down into a squatting position. Descend slowly over 3 seconds all the way down but not to bounce as this will decrease the effectiveness of the workout. Then come back up over 1 second, squeeze the buttock and thigh muscles for 1 second and then continue the repetitions. While descending, the arms should be slowly raised forward for balance. Matt does not count repetitions for this; rather he does this non-stop for a full minute.

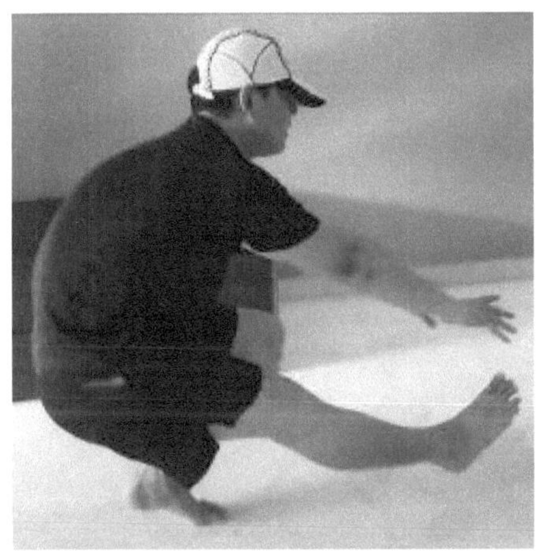

Figure 3b. Pistol squats. This takes the form of a pistol on full descend, hence the name. This is a single leg squat. The other leg is left in full extension with heel above the ground. At no time should the heel of this leg touch the ground. Matt initially had to hold on to a chair for balance. After a while, he could balance with his two arms outstretched.

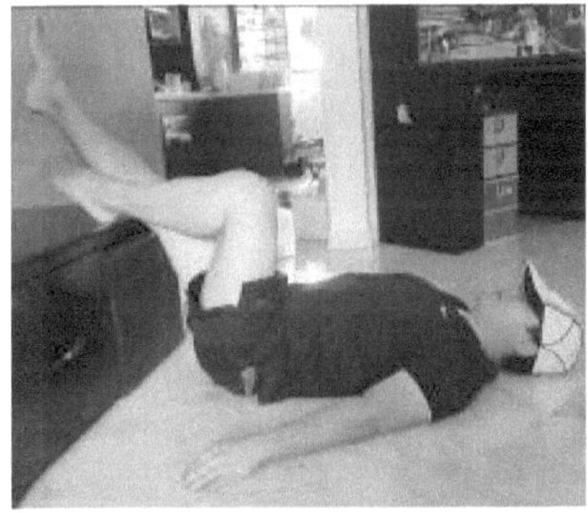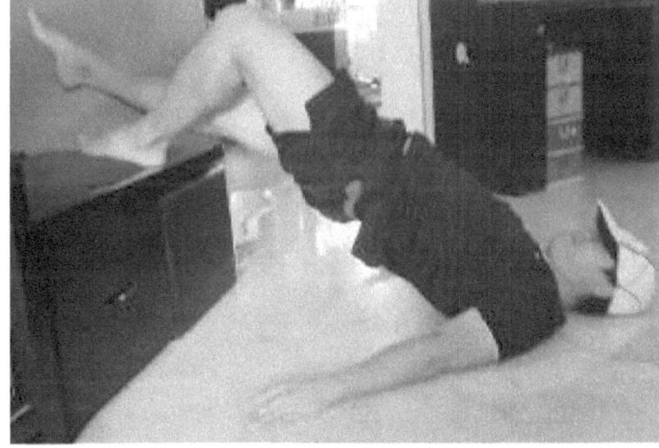

Figure 3c. Bridges. This works more of the hamstrings and gluteus muscles. Lie back down on the floor, soles of the feet on the ground. Matt keeps his feet elevated on a coffee-table to increase the intensity. Use the heel to push down onto the table or ground to lift the buttock up till full extension of the hip. Then squeeze the hamstrings and buttock muscles at the top. Like the pistol squat extend the leg not being exercised with the heel just above but not touching the ground or coffee-table.

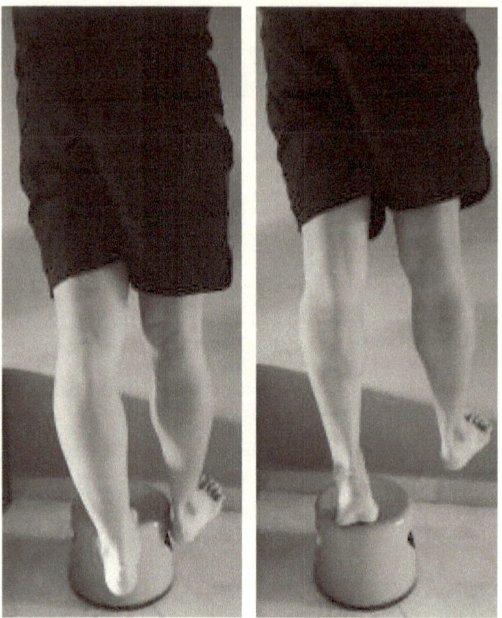

Figure 3d. Calf raises. For this calf muscle workout, start by standing on one leg. Push down using the ball of the foot and raise the heel off the ground to achieve a full calf contraction. Squeeze the calf at the top, hold then slowly the heel to the ground and repeat the repetition. Matt uses a sitting stool to get a better range of motion. The ball of the foot is placed on the step while the heel is left free. This allows the heel to descend to achieve a full stretch.

Matt does one set of the Pistol squats which are quickly followed by Bridges then the Calf raises – this constitutes one full set. This way of grouping two or more exercises without rest into one set is called a 'superset'. The exercises can be of the same or different muscle group. This differs from the 'drop-set' whereby the intensity is dropped instead.

In summary

.)   One minute of regular squats

.i)   Matt does 5 sets of the Pistol squats – Bridges – Calf raises with a 2 minute rest in
between sets.

.ii)   Matt finishes off his Day 3 exercise by either skipping rope for or short bursts of
50 metre sprints for a total of 15 minutes.

Days 4, 5 and 6 are just a duplicate of Days 1, 2 and 3. Matt does not have an
exercise routine on Day 7. However Matt tries to practise some technique skills
that day. Currently Matt is working on his – front lever, hand stands, planche and
muscle ups.

Front lever – where one holds onto the pull-up bar and holds the entire trunk and
legs horizontally (this is a form of static exercise).

Hand stands – where one 'stands' on both hands with the body held vertically.
This can later be progressed on to hand stand push-ups to work on the shoulders
using the body's entire weight.

Planche – sort of the opposite of the front lever. The trunk and legs are held
horizontally above the ground supported only by the arms.

Muscle ups – a combination of the pull-up and dip but with a difference in
technique. Instead of a pull-up, the body is swung upwards more forcefully into a
dip position and completed with a dip.

These are cool exercises. However they require quite a bit of core strength and coordination with balance. They have easier variations such as the tuck and straddle prior to the exercise proper. Still a work in progress for Matt!

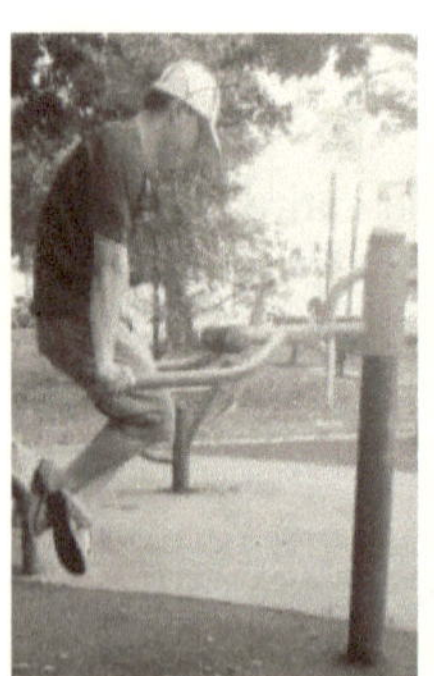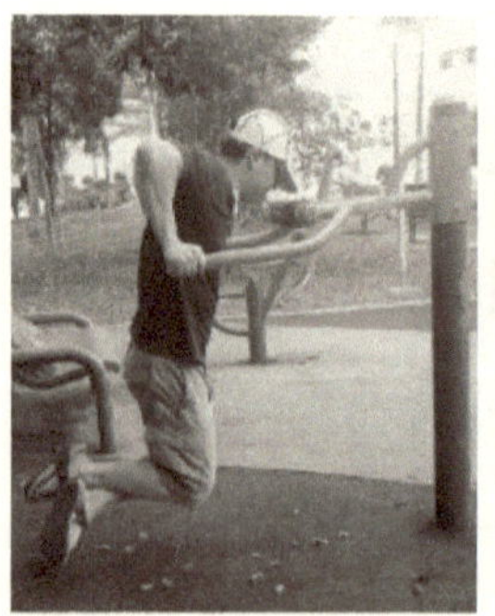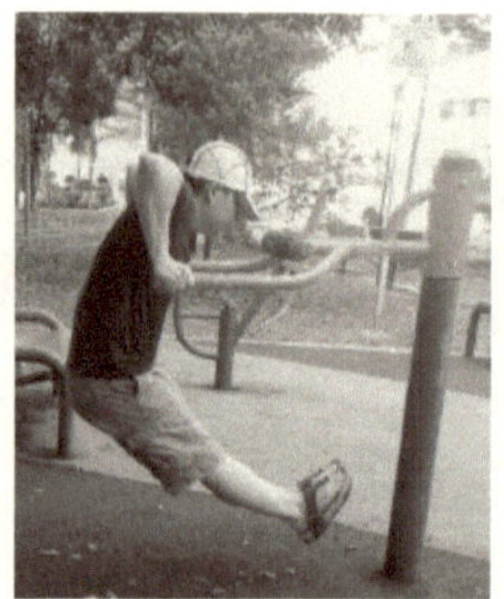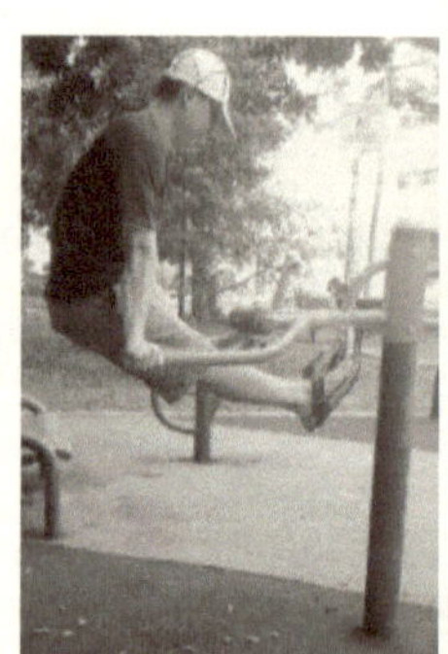

Figure 4. The dip.

Progression – using weights, leverage and stability

There are a few ways to increase or decrease the intensity of the exercise as shown in the previous chapter. However I thought that it would be good to equip you with the principles so that you can make the adjustments yourself.

Weights

The most obvious actually would be adding external weights to your body. Although no longer purely relying on your own bodyweight. It is a method to take your game to the next level. There are plenty of ways to do this.

Some are products specially made for this purpose:

1) Weighted body vest: this is worn like a vest or jacket and contains weights

2) Weight belt: this is worn like a belt and has a metal chain to attach barbell weights to the belt – useful in weighted pull-ups, dips or muscle ups

3) Metal chains which function like the belt but placed around the neck without the weights

Some can be self-made:

1) Carrying a backpack with weights, heavy books or bottles filled with water or sand. This goes well with pull-ups, push-ups and dips.

2) Similarly carrying your young kid on your back serves as an excellent external weight while having some fun with your kid – they always find it exciting.

Leverage

The root word of leverage is lever. My physics teacher used to teach me about using levers to ease the work of doing everyday things. One good example is the wheelbarrow. The weight is in the middle of where the wheel and handles are. As the distance from the wheel to the handles is greater than that of the distance from the wheel to the weight, less force is needed to carry the weight. In calisthenics the same principle is applied by adjusting the effective length of the legs. By bending the legs at the knees and/or hips or by spreading the legs, this length is shortened and vice versa. A good example would be doing push-ups on the knees which are easier than on the toes. To make the push-up harder, one can simply raise the height of the feet higher than that of the hands. This decreases the amount of weight supported by the feet and throws the balance over to the upper limbs. The higher the height of the feet in proportion to that of the hands, the greater the amount borne.

Stability

Bringing instability into the picture causes the muscles to work harder. This is to keep the body in equilibrium to avoid falling over. Overall, makes for a better exercise. For example, while doing the push-up one can place the feet on a Swiss ball instead of on the ground. As the ball tends to roll in all directions, the entire body needs to work harder to maintain balance. The same is true if suspended rings were used for a push-up or pull-ups. Imagine holding on to suspended rings which tend to swing in all directions while you are doing the pull-up or push-up. The muscles not only need to work on lifting or pushing the body, they also need o work on preventing the rings from swinging away. In short, fatiguing the muscles easier and intensifying the exercise.

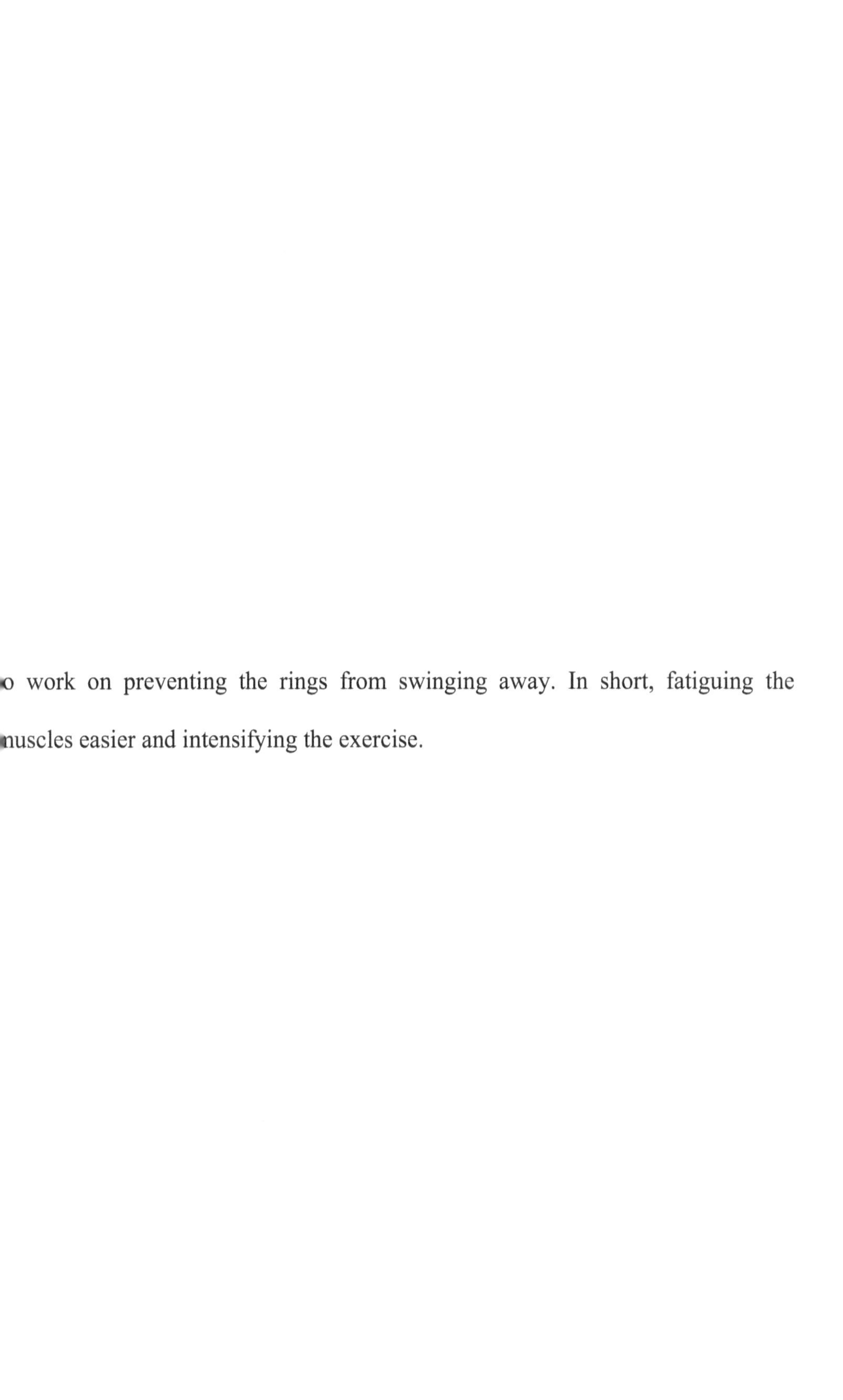

Improve your results – 'TACT, M'

Track your performance. Measure it!

In school our teachers would see how much we understood a topic by giving us a test at the end of every semester. They would also calculate the average of the class and tell us how we were doing in comparison to our classmates. At work companies have key performance indicators (KPIs) to gauge our productivity and work contribution (directly affecting our bonus!). How about for your exercise programme? How do we know we are improving?

Try this:

i) Have a diary on your progress in terms of repetitions and progressions. This would keep you more motivated and goal-driven to do the exercise, to do the extra repetition, to bear with the burn. If you find yourself stagnating for a long time, go back to the basic principles – make sure that you are not neglecting them.

ii) If your goal is weight loss, you may then use weight as the parameter. However do note that muscle has weight and as one gains muscle mass, the body mass index (BMI = kg/m²) also increases. A more accurate measure would then be the percentage body fat. There are a few ways to measure this and can be found on the internet. But as more fat is lost the body gets better sculpted and muscles more defined. Again the internet has a series of pictures for each range of estimated percentage body fat. One point to note, Matt discovered that fat distribution is genetically determined. Body fat is lost throughout the body when there is a calorie deficit and not only a specific part of the body. Fat, however is lost in some areas faster than others. So do not expect the tummy fat to disappear just because one is constantly doing abdominal exercises. To lose fat, one needs to be in calorie deficit. As mentioned, this gets easier with a greater muscle mass and metabolism. I do apologise for side-tracking. In short, what does not get measured, does not get improved.

Adhere to the basic principles

This is worth reiterating. I would encourage you to re-read the topic 'some basic principles' above. With these guiding principles you will have a sturdy foundation on which to build your programme on.

Consistency

To be successful in anything in life we need to put in the hours. For the busy professional this may be difficult. I am not saying that we need to put in a lot of time for each routine. Matt does not take more than 30 minutes for of his workout sessions. In addition he saves time as he does not need to travel for his exercise for his push and leg days. He does need to take a 2 minute walk down to a nearby playground for his pull days as he needs a pull-up bar. You can always get a pull-up bar at home which can be attached to your door-frame to cut down on your time even more. What I actually mean is that we must not stop! Be consistent! We busy professionals may not have the luxury of time per day. But we can always allocate 30 minutes every day. An hour might be difficult to squeeze out of a day but 30 minutes is not that difficult – cut down on television time, movies and snoozing the alarm-clock. This done regularly over time is manifold better than 2 hours on end and then pausing for a few months or stopping altogether.

Try this:

a)   Schedule it. Create a routine.

i)   Things that do not get scheduled do not get done. Put it down on your phone calendar. Set a time for it so when the time comes your subconscious will be nagging you to do it.

ii)   After a while once you have figured out where to best place this 30 minutes of blocked out time, create and stick to that routine. You might then not need to schedule it anymore and it will become more of a habit rather than a task to do. You never schedule when to brush your teeth at 5am and then again at 10pm, you just know subconsciously that it needs to get done. Whatever time, whatever plan it may be you will eventually figure it out as long as you schedule it initially.

b)   Don't make excuses. Just start.

We can always make excuses. There are so many reasons to not exercise. I have no time. I am too tired. I need to do the housework. I need to look after the kids. By the time you are done thinking of your excuse, Matt has just completed his workout session in the same time – just an exaggeration. The point is you should not spend too much time fighting in your head.

Try this:

i)   Create that habit. We are what we repeatedly do. Once the scheduled time has arrived or the kids have just gone to bed or you have just woken up, just get down and start doing your push-ups. Complete your first set then you can continue your fight in your head during your rest period then go down again. The excuses eventually faded and soon Matt found it weird or incomplete if he does not do his exercises. Subconsciously Matt feels that it is just not right and something has not been done when he does not exercise or when he does not brush his teeth or make the bed.

ii)   Make it a priority. Matt has made regular exercise a high priority on his list of things to do. Indeed, the beginning is always the hardest. That is the time when you are still adjusting your routine, finding that common ground in terms of allocating time for your daily priorities. That is the time when Matt still had a lot of internal struggles. However what helped was the 'Why'. Matt thought of exercise as an investment. We invest in our family, work, friends, real estate and stocks. But how about you? Investing in you. Invest in your health. This is also

part of self-development like education, to better your work prospects and skills.
Higher energy levels for work and family. Less neck and back pains. Normal
cholesterol and blood pressure level. Hopefully a longer and more meaningful life.
By placing greater importance it gets done.

Take a break

But I thought that we must be consistent? Yes, but every few months it is good to
take one or two weeks off your exercise regime to avoid burnout and stagnation.
Weight-lifting be it bodyweight or external weights can take a toll on the body.
Muscle accommodates and heals pretty fast. But the tendons, joints and ligaments
do not. Matt found that after pounding consistently he had some pain in his
tendons and joints. Carrying his baby at home every day did not help either. A one
or two weeks' break allowed his body to catch up on some recovery and
strengthening of the non-muscle tissues. Depending on the intensity of the
exercise, this break can be every 4 to 6 months. Matt takes a break every 6 months
but still goes for a light swim with his children and light jog when he brings his
older two daughters to the park to cycle. It does not have to be a total break. You
could still go for a swim or a slow jog if you wanted to. After two weeks of rest
Matt was able to do more repetitions and progressed better. Matt could also
withstand the burn longer.

Make it fun, challenge yourself!

Matt likes to do a few variations for his routines. But he only does a set each. This keeps it interesting and fun as there is a constant change throughout the workout session. If you have the time and would prefer to give your muscles the extra burn, you can perform 3-5 sets for each variation. Matt likes to keep his exercise routines to about 30 minutes and then he is done and back to his daily chores.

Drop-sets. Matt does a lot of drop-sets which involve working a muscle to failure, and then reducing the intensity before immediately continuing. In calisthenics the intensity is changed by changing the leverage or if there is an external weight like using a belt or vest, removing it. This enhances time under tension and metabolic stress which encourages muscle to grow. Another way to look at time under tension is the total work done. Metabolic stress increases with the accumulation of metabolic waste products i.e. lactic acid and inorganic phosphates; basically fatiguing the muscle as much as possible prior to allowing it to rest.

Super-sets. This is another way to enhance the metabolic stress and time under tension whilst being time-efficient. This is way of grouping two or more exercises without rest into one set is called a 'superset'. The exercises can be of the same or different muscle group; largely divided into two types:

Antagonist-agonist supersets

The agonist muscle is the muscle which undergoes contraction while the antagonist muscle is the one which relaxes. When flexing the elbow, the biceps contracts and hence is the agonist and the triceps relaxes i.e. the antagonist muscle.

So a superset of this kind would be like doing a push-up quickly followed by a chin-up for example.

Compound supersets

This type uses the same body part in a successive manner. A good example would be doing a dip then a push-up.

Cheat repetitions. These are improper and incomplete repetitions; repetitions performed with some amount of momentum (swinging). But I thought we are not supposed to do that? Yes cheat repetitions are done using poor technique. You only start doing it once you have achieved failure for a particular set. Then you continue performing repetitions despite improper form because your muscles are too fatigued. The theory behind it is in doing so you stimulate more motor units and increase the metabolic stress. A good tip would be to still squeeze at the top of whatever range contraction you can achieve and go slow on the negatives like normal repetitions. Another tip would be to just concentrate on your breathing – in and out; as by now your muscles will be burning like mad.

At least every 6 months (sometimes even monthly), Matt changes the sequence or structure of his routine just to confuse the muscles a little. There is no hard and fast rule, no 'correct' or 'wrong' way.

This is Matt's favourite routine:

Day 1 - Back and biceps

Day 2 – Chest, shoulders, triceps

Day 3 – Legs

Day 4 – Back and biceps

Day 5 – Chest, shoulders, triceps

Day 6 - Legs

Day 7 – Rest

Another routine he does:

Day 1 – Chest and back

Day 2 – Shoulders and legs

Day 3 – Rest

Day 4 – Chest and back

Day 5 – Shoulders and legs

Day 6 – Rest

Day 7 – Sprints and skipping

Day 1 and 4:

Archer pull-ups → regular pull-ups → chin-ups → Australian pull-ups →Rest for 1 minute → Decline Archer push-ups → Decline push-ups → regular push-ups → push-ups on knees → Rest for 2 minutes then repeat again for a total of 3 sets

Day 2 and 5:

Pike push-ups feet elevated → regular Pike push-ups → Rest 1 minute → Pistol-squats → Bridges → Calf raises → regular squats for 1 minute → Rest 2 minutes then repeat for a total of 3 sets

Yet another routine:

Day 1 - Back and biceps

Day 2 – Chest, shoulders, triceps

Day 3 – Legs

Day 4 – Back and biceps

Day 5 – Chest, shoulders, triceps

Day 6 - Legs

Day 7 – Rest

Similar to Matt's favourite routine but the variations are tweaked a little.

Day 1 and 4:

Pull-ups → One-arm Australian pull-ups → Australian pull-ups → Rest for 2 minutes then repeat to complete 5 sets

Day 2 and 5:

Archer push-ups → push-ups → push-ups on knees → Rest for 2 minutes then repeat to complete 5 sets

Day 6:

Skipping for 15minutes

Pistol squats → Bridges → Calf raises → One minute squats → Rest for 2 minutes then repeat to complete 5 sets

Calisthenics training is fun and very versatile. You can design and mix-and-match your own routines. However the most important thing is to master the basics principles and techniques well. Matt is still at an early stage of his journey. There are still some advanced techniques like the front lever, hand stands, planche and muscle ups which are works in progress. Though the basic exercises is already sufficient, Matt finds these advance techniques fun and challenging. Whatever your 'Why' is, we wish you all the best in your journey!

Track your performance

Adhere to the basic principles

Consistency

Take a break

Make it fun, challenge yourself!